No
THE POWER OF LETTING GO

A Journey to inner peace and personal transformation

MELISSA J. POWELL

TABLE OF CONTENT

INTRODUCTION

The Concept of Letting Go

Why Letting Go is Empowering

How This Book Will Help You

In a world that often glorifies control, achievement, and relentless pursuit, the concept of letting go can seem counterintuitive almost like surrendering. Yet, there is a profound power in releasing what no longer serves us. Letting go is not about giving up; it is about freeing ourselves from the invisible chains that hold us back, whether they are past regrets, toxic relationships, unrealistic expectations, or self-doubt. It is an act of courage, an assertion that our worth and happiness are not defined by what we hold onto, but by what we are willing to release.

Why is letting go so empowering? Because it returns the control to you not over circumstances, but over your own mind and emotions. When we let go, we break free from the constant mental chatter, the what-ifs, and the should-haves. We create space for new possibilities, for growth, and for peace. It is in this space that true transformation happens, where you are no longer a prisoner of your past or a victim of your fears, but a creator of your present and future.

This book is your guide on this transformative journey. It will show you how to identify what you need to let go of and provide you with the tools to do so. Through practical advice, personal stories, and powerful exercises, you will learn how to release what is weighing you down and embrace the freedom and empowerment that come with letting go. Whether it's fear, guilt, or the need for approval, you will discover how to unburden yourself and live a life of greater authenticity, joy, and purpose.

Letting go is not just an act; it's a mindset, a way of being. This book will help you cultivate that mindset and, in doing so, unlock a life that is lighter, freer, and more aligned with who you truly are.

CHAPTER 1

Understanding Attachment

The Nature of Attachment

Emotional and Mental Clutter

The Cost of Holding On

Understanding Attachment

Attachment is a fundamental aspect of the human experience. It shapes our relationships, influences our decisions, and often dictates the quality of our emotional and mental well-being. At its core, attachment is the deep emotional bond that connects us to other people, objects, ideas, or outcomes. While attachment is natural and necessary, it can also lead to emotional and mental clutter when it becomes unhealthy or excessive. Understanding the nature of attachment, recognizing its impact on our lives, and learning how to manage it can empower us to lead more fulfilling lives.

The Nature of Attachment

What is Attachment?

Attachment is a complex and multi-faceted concept rooted in our biological and psychological makeup. It refers to the emotional bond that forms between individuals, often starting in infancy with the relationship between a child and their primary caregiver. This early attachment plays a crucial role in shaping our future relationships and emotional health.

The study of attachment gained prominence with the work of British psychologist John Bowlby, who developed Attachment Theory. Bowlby argued that the bonds we form in our early years have a profound impact on our emotional development and behavior throughout life. According to Bowlby, attachment behaviors are biologically driven, ensuring that infants stay close to their caregivers for protection and survival.

Attachment Theory identifies four primary attachment styles: Secure, Anxious, Avoidant, and Disorganized. Each style represents a different way of relating to others based on our early experiences:

Secure Attachment: Individuals with a secure attachment style tend to have healthy, trusting relationships.

They feel comfortable with intimacy and are generally confident in their ability to handle challenges.

Anxious Attachment: People with an anxious attachment style often crave closeness and approval but fear abandonment. They may become overly dependent on others and struggle with insecurity.

Avoidant Attachment: Those with an avoidant attachment style may distance themselves emotionally from others. They often value independence and self-sufficiency, sometimes at the expense of deep connections.

Disorganized Attachment: This style is characterized by a lack of clear attachment behavior. Individuals may display a mix of anxious and avoidant tendencies, often resulting from trauma or inconsistent caregiving in childhood.

These attachment styles serve as the blueprint for how we approach relationships, handle stress, and navigate the world around us. Understanding our attachment style can help us recognize patterns in our behavior and make more conscious choices in our relationships.

Why Do We Form Attachments?

Attachment is not just a psychological concept; it has deep evolutionary and biological roots. From an evolutionary perspective, attachment behaviors have developed to ensure the survival of the species. In the early stages of human development, infants who stayed close to their caregivers were more likely to survive, as they were protected from predators and received the necessary care and nourishment.

Biologically, the formation of attachments is closely linked to the brain's reward system. When we form a bond with someone, our brain releases neurotransmitters like oxytocin and dopamine, which promote feelings of pleasure, trust, and bonding. This chemical reinforcement encourages us to seek out and maintain close relationships.

Beyond survival, attachment plays a crucial role in our emotional well-being. Healthy attachments provide us with a sense of security, belonging, and support. They help us navigate the ups and downs of life, offering comfort during difficult times and joy during moments of connection.

However, not all attachments are created equal. While some attachments enhance our lives, others can become sources of stress, anxiety, and emotional pain. The key to understanding attachment lies in recognizing the difference between healthy and unhealthy bonds.

Healthy vs. Unhealthy Attachments

Healthy attachments are characterized by mutual respect, trust, and emotional support. They allow for independence and growth while providing a secure base from which we can explore the world. In healthy relationships, there is a balance between closeness and individuality, and both parties feel valued and understood.

Unhealthy attachments, on the other hand, are often rooted in fear, insecurity, or a need for control. These attachments can manifest as dependency, jealousy, or an inability to let go. They may lead to patterns of behavior that are detrimental to our emotional and mental health, such as clinging to toxic relationships, holding onto past hurts, or becoming overly attached to material possessions.

Understanding the nature of our attachments and distinguishing between healthy and unhealthy bonds is the first step toward achieving emotional and mental well-being. By cultivating healthy attachments and letting go of those that no longer serve us, we can create a more balanced and fulfilling life.

Emotional and Mental Clutter

What is Emotional and Mental Clutter?

Emotional and mental clutter refers to the accumulation of unresolved feelings, thoughts, and attachments that weigh us down and prevent us from living fully in the present. This clutter can manifest in various ways, such as lingering resentments, unfulfilled desires, or a constant preoccupation with the past or future.

When we hold onto emotional and mental clutter, it creates a psychological burden that affects our overall well-being. Just as physical clutter in our environment can create stress and overwhelm, emotional and mental clutter can lead to anxiety, depression, and a diminished quality of life.

Attachment plays a significant role in the accumulation of emotional and mental clutter. Our attachments to people, memories, and outcomes can create a web of unresolved emotions and thoughts that clutter our minds and hearts. Understanding how attachment contributes to this clutter is essential for finding clarity and peace.

Attachment and Emotional Clutter

Emotional clutter often stems from our attachments to past experiences, relationships, and unresolved emotions. When we become attached to certain outcomes or hold onto memories of past hurts, we create a mental and emotional residue that lingers in our minds.

For example, consider someone who has experienced a painful breakup. If they remain attached to the idea of the relationship or the person they were with, they may find it difficult to move on. This attachment can lead to emotional clutter in the form of lingering sadness, anger, or longing. These unresolved emotions can affect their ability to form new relationships or fully engage with the present.

Similarly, attachment to material possessions can create emotional clutter. When we attach our sense of identity or self-worth to the things we own, we may find ourselves overwhelmed by the need to acquire more or by the fear of losing what we have. This attachment can lead to feelings of inadequacy, jealousy, or dissatisfaction, creating a cycle of emotional clutter.

Letting go of these attachments requires a conscious effort to process and release unresolved emotions. By acknowledging and addressing our emotional clutter, we can create space for new experiences and healthier attachments.

Attachment and Mental Clutter

Mental clutter is the cognitive load that results from holding onto unhealthy attachments. It includes repetitive thoughts, worries, and overthinking that occupy our mental space and prevent us from focusing on what truly matters.

CHAPTER 2

Identifying What No Longer Serves You

Recognizing Negative Patterns

Toxic Relationships and Situations

Outdated Beliefs and Habits

Identifying what no longer serves you is a crucial step in personal growth and transformation. We often hold onto patterns, relationships, and beliefs that were once helpful but now hinder our progress. This chapter evaluates deep into the process of recognizing these elements in our lives, understanding their impact, and taking the necessary steps to release them.

Recognizing Negative Patterns

Negative patterns are recurrent behaviors, thoughts, or emotions that sabotage our well-being. They are often rooted in past experiences, traumas, or learned behaviors and become ingrained over time. These patterns can manifest in various areas of our lives, including relationships, work, and personal development.

Common Negative Patterns

1. Self-Sabotage: Engaging in behaviors that prevent success or personal fulfillment.

2. Procrastination: Delaying tasks, leading to stress and missed opportunities.

3. Perfectionism: Setting unattainable standards, leading to frustration and burnout.

4. People-Pleasing: Prioritizing others' needs at the expense of your own well-being.

5. Negative Self-Talk: Internal dialogue that reinforces self-doubt and low self-esteem.

Identifying Your Negative Patterns

To identify your negative patterns, start by observing your thoughts, behaviors, and emotional responses. Journaling can be an effective tool to track these patterns over time. Pay attention to situations where you feel stuck, frustrated, or overwhelmed. Ask yourself:

What triggers these feelings?

How do I respond to these triggers?

What recurring thoughts or behaviors do I notice?

By answering these questions, you can begin to uncover the negative patterns that no longer serve you.

The Impact of Negative Patterns

Negative patterns can have a profound impact on your life, leading to stress, anxiety, and a sense of unfulfillment. They can hinder personal and professional growth, strain relationships, and perpetuate a cycle of negativity. Recognizing these patterns is the first step toward breaking free from their grip and creating positive change.

Breaking Free from Negative Patterns

Breaking free from negative patterns requires self-awareness, commitment, and patience. Start by acknowledging the patterns and their impact on your life. Then, set clear intentions to change these behaviors. Practice mindfulness and self-compassion as you steer this process. Consider seeking support from a therapist, coach, or support group to help you stay accountable and motivated.

Toxic Relationships and Situation

Toxic relationships are those that drain your energy, undermine your self-worth, and create emotional or psychological harm. They can occur in various forms, including romantic relationships, friendships, family dynamics, and work environments. These relationships are often characterized by manipulation, control, and a lack of respect or empathy.

Signs of a Toxic Relationship

1. Constant Criticism: One or both parties regularly criticize, belittle, or undermine each other.

2. Manipulation: One person uses guilt, fear, or other tactics to control or influence the other.

3. Lack of Support: The relationship lacks mutual support, with one person feeling neglected or unimportant.

4. High Conflict: Frequent arguments, tension, and unresolved issues dominate the relationship.

5. Emotional Drain: The relationship leaves you feeling exhausted, anxious, or depressed.

Identifying Toxic Situations

Toxic situations are environments or circumstances that negatively impact your mental, emotional, or physical well-being. These can include toxic work environments, unhealthy family dynamics, or social settings that promote negative behaviors.

Signs of a Toxic Situation

1. Chronic Stress: The situation consistently causes stress, anxiety, or fear.

2. Lack of Boundaries: Boundaries are not respected, leading to feelings of violation or discomfort.

3. Unhealthy Competition: The environment fosters unhealthy competition, jealousy, or resentment.

4. Gossip and Negativity: The atmosphere is filled with gossip, negativity, and backstabbing.

5. Feeling Trapped: You feel stuck or unable to escape the situation, leading to a sense of hopelessness.

The Impact of Toxic Relationships and Situations

Toxic relationships and situations can have a devastating impact on your mental, emotional, and physical health. They can lead to chronic stress, anxiety, depression, and even physical illness. These environments can also erode your self-esteem, confidence, and sense of identity.

How to Distance Yourself from Toxic Relationships and Situations

1. Set Boundaries: Clearly define and communicate your boundaries. This may involve limiting contact, saying no, or distancing yourself from the toxic person or situation.

2. Seek Support: Reach out to trusted friends, family members, or professionals for support and guidance.

3. Focus on Self-Care: Prioritize your well-being by engaging in activities that nourish your mind, body, and soul.

4. Let Go of Guilt: Recognize that you have the right to protect yourself from

harm and that it's okay to prioritize your health and happiness.

5. Make a Plan: Create a plan to gradually remove yourself from the toxic relationship or situation. This may involve finding a new job, ending a relationship, or seeking therapy.

Outdated Beliefs and Habits

Outdated beliefs are long-held convictions that no longer align with your current values, goals, or circumstances. These beliefs may have served a purpose in the past but now hinder your growth and prevent you from achieving your full potential.

Common Outdated Beliefs

1. I'm Not Good Enough: A belief rooted in self-doubt and low self-esteem.

2. Success Means Sacrifice: The idea that achieving success requires suffering or giving up what you love.

3. I Must Follow Tradition: A belief that you must adhere to cultural or family traditions, even if they no longer resonate with you.

4. Change is Dangerous: The fear that change will lead to negative consequences.

5. I Must Please Others: The belief that your worth is determined by how much you please others.

Identifying Your Outdated Beliefs

To identify your outdated beliefs, reflect on your current goals and values. Ask yourself:

What beliefs do I hold that no longer align with my current values or goals?

How do these beliefs limit my growth or potential?

Are these beliefs based on past experiences, societal norms, or family expectations?

Journaling and introspection can help you uncover these beliefs and understand their origins.

Understanding Outdated Habits

Outdated habits are behaviors or routines that once served a purpose but now hinder your progress. These habits can be physical, such as unhealthy eating or lack of exercise, or mental, such as negative thinking patterns or procrastination.

Common Outdated Habits

1. Procrastination: Delaying tasks that are essential for growth or success.

2. Overworking: Working excessively to the detriment of your health and personal life.

3. Negative Self-Talk: Engaging in self-criticism and doubt.

4. Avoiding Challenges: Avoiding new opportunities or challenges out of fear of failure.

5. Clinging to Comfort Zones: Staying within familiar routines and avoiding change.

The Impact of Outdated Beliefs and Habits

Outdated beliefs and habits can hold you back from achieving your full potential. They create mental and emotional barriers that prevent you from pursuing your dreams and living authentically. These beliefs and habits can also lead to feelings of frustration, stagnation, and dissatisfaction.

How to Release Outdated Beliefs and Habits

1. Challenge Your Beliefs: Question the validity of your outdated beliefs. Are they based on facts or assumptions? How do they limit you?

2. Embrace Change: Recognize that change is a natural part of growth and that letting go of outdated beliefs and habits can lead to new opportunities.

3. Adopt New Perspectives: Replace outdated beliefs with new, empowering ones that align with your current values and goals.

4. Create New Habits: Develop new habits that support your growth and well-being. Start small and gradually build on your progress.

5. Practice Self-Compassion: Be kind to yourself as you navigate this process. Letting go of long-held beliefs and habits can be challenging, but it's a necessary step toward personal growth.

Therefore identifying what no longer serves you is a powerful step toward personal transformation. By recognizing and releasing negative patterns, toxic relationships and situations, and outdated beliefs and habits, you create space for new opportunities, growth, and fulfillment. Remember that this process requires self-awareness, courage, and patience. As you let go of what no longer serves you, you pave the way for a more authentic, empowered, and joyful life

CHAPTER 3

The Psychology of Letting Go

The Fear of the Unknown.

Overcoming Resistance to Change

Releasing Emotional Baggage

Letting go is a profound act that often lies at the heart of personal growth and transformation. Whether it's releasing past trauma, moving on from a toxic relationship, or simply discarding outdated beliefs, letting go is essential to embracing a healthier, more fulfilling life. However, the process is rarely easy. It requires confronting deep-seated fears, overcoming resistance, and freeing oneself from the emotional baggage that often weighs us down.

The psychology of letting go encompasses understanding the mental and emotional mechanisms that keep us attached to what no longer serves us. It involves recognizing the fears that arise when facing the unknown, addressing the resistance to change that naturally occurs, and learning how to release the emotional burdens that keep us stuck in place.

In this section, we will explore these three critical aspects of the letting go process. We will look into the fear of the unknown, examine the nature of resistance to change, and provide strategies for releasing emotional baggage. By understanding these psychological barriers, we can begin to dismantle them and move toward a life of greater freedom and peace.

The Fear of the Unknown

The fear of the unknown is one of the most powerful psychological barriers to letting go. This fear stems from the human brain's natural inclination toward familiarity and certainty. When faced with the prospect of change, the mind often conjures worst-case scenarios, fueling anxiety and making it difficult to move forward.

The Comfort of Certainty

Humans are wired to seek out stability and predictability. From an evolutionary standpoint, our ancestors relied on predictable patterns for survival—knowing where to find food, recognizing threats, and understanding social hierarchies. This need for certainty is deeply ingrained in our psychology and influences our behavior even today.

When we cling to what we know, even if it's harmful or unfulfilling, it's often because the alternative—stepping into the unknown—feels far more frightening. The unknown represents potential risks, and the human brain, in its quest to protect us, often overestimates these risks. As a result, we become paralyzed by fear, preferring the devil we know over the uncertainty of what might be.

The Illusion of Control

Another factor that contributes to the fear of the unknown is the illusion of control. When we hold on to the familiar, we believe we have some level of control over our lives. This belief can be comforting, even if it's not entirely accurate. The reality is that much of life is beyond our control, and clinging to false certainties can prevent us from embracing new opportunities and experiences.

Letting go requires surrendering this illusion of control and accepting that uncertainty is an inherent part of life. This acceptance can be challenging, as it involves acknowledging our vulnerability and the unpredictability of the future. However, it is also liberating, as it frees us from the need to micromanage every aspect of our lives.

The Role of Anxiety

Anxiety is a natural response to the unknown. When faced with uncertainty, the mind tends to catastrophize, imagining worst-case scenarios and amplifying fears. This anxiety can be overwhelming, leading to avoidance behaviors that keep us stuck in familiar patterns, even when those patterns are detrimental to our well-being.

One way to combat anxiety related to the unknown is through mindfulness and grounding techniques. By staying present and focusing on what we can control in the moment, we can reduce the power of anxiety and make more informed, less fear-driven decisions. Additionally, reframing uncertainty as an opportunity for growth rather than a threat can help shift our mindset and reduce fear.

Embracing Uncertainty

Embracing uncertainty is a crucial step in the process of letting go. It involves shifting our perspective from fear to curiosity, recognizing that the unknown is not inherently dangerous but full of potential. By viewing the unknown as a blank canvas rather than a dark void, we can begin to see the possibilities that lie ahead.

One practical approach to embracing uncertainty is to gradually expose ourselves to new experiences. By taking small steps outside our comfort zone, we can build confidence and reduce the fear associated with the unknown. Over time, these small steps can lead to significant personal growth and a greater sense of freedom.

Overcoming Resistance to Change

Resistance to change is another major obstacle in the process of letting go. This resistance can manifest in various forms, including procrastination, self-sabotage, and a stubborn attachment to the status quo. Understanding the roots of this resistance and learning how to overcome it is essential for personal transformation.

The Psychology of Resistance

At its core, resistance to change is rooted in fear—fear of failure, fear of loss, and fear of the unknown. The human brain is designed to conserve energy and avoid risk, which is why it often resists change, even when change is necessary for growth. This resistance is often unconscious, manifesting as excuses, rationalizations, and avoidance behaviors that keep us from taking action.

One way to understand resistance is through the concept of cognitive dissonance. Cognitive dissonance occurs when our actions are inconsistent with our beliefs or values, creating psychological discomfort. To reduce this discomfort, we may resist change by rationalizing our current behavior or avoiding situations that challenge our beliefs.

For example, if we believe that we should leave a toxic relationship but feel unable to do so, we may experience cognitive dissonance. To resolve this discomfort, we might convince ourselves that the relationship isn't as bad as it seems or that we're not ready to leave. This rationalization helps reduce the discomfort of cognitive dissonance but ultimately keeps us stuck.

The Role of Habit

Habits play a significant role in resistance to change. When we engage in the same behaviors repeatedly, they become ingrained in our neural pathways, making them automatic and difficult to break. These habits provide a sense of familiarity and comfort, even if they're not serving our best interests.

Breaking free from ingrained habits requires conscious effort and persistence. It involves recognizing the triggers that lead to habitual behaviors and replacing them with new, healthier habits. This process can be challenging, as it requires rewiring the brain and stepping out of our comfort zone.

One effective strategy for overcoming habitual resistance is to start small. Rather than attempting to make sweeping changes all at once, focus on making incremental adjustments that are more manageable. Over time, these small changes can lead to significant shifts in behavior and mindset.

The Influence of Identity

Our sense of identity is closely tied to our resistance to change. We often resist letting go because it threatens our self-concept—our understanding of who we are. For example, if we identify as someone who is strong and independent, we may resist asking for help or admitting vulnerability, even when it's in our best interest.

Letting go often requires redefining our identity and embracing new aspects of ourselves. This process can be uncomfortable, as it involves letting go of old narratives and beliefs that no longer serve us. However, it is also an opportunity for growth and self-discovery.

One way to overcome identity-based resistance is to focus on the aspects of our identity that are flexible and adaptable. By recognizing that we are not defined by any one trait or belief, we can begin to explore new possibilities and expand our self-concept.

Strategies for Overcoming Resistance

Overcoming resistance to change requires a combination of self-awareness, persistence, and compassion. Here are some strategies to help navigate this process:

1. Self-Reflection: Take time to reflect on the areas of your life where you

feel resistance. What fears or beliefs are holding you back? By identifying these underlying factors, you can begin to address them more effectively.

2. Mindfulness: Practice mindfulness to stay present and aware of your thoughts and emotions. This awareness can help you recognize when resistance is arising and give you the space to choose a different response.

3. Positive Reinforcement: Reward yourself for taking small steps toward change. Positive reinforcement can help build momentum and reduce resistance over time.

4. Support Systems: Surround yourself with supportive individuals who encourage your growth. Having a strong support system can help you

stay motivated and accountable during the process of change.

5. Compassion: Be gentle with yourself as you navigate resistance. Change is difficult, and it's natural to encounter setbacks along the way. Practice self-compassion and remind yourself that growth is a gradual process.

Releasing Emotional Baggage

Emotional baggage refers to the unresolved emotions, traumas, and negative experiences that we carry with us from the past. This baggage can weigh us down, preventing us from fully engaging with the present and moving forward in our lives. Releasing emotional baggage is a crucial step in the process of letting go, as it allows us to free ourselves

from the past and create space for
new experiences.

Understanding Emotional Baggage

Emotional baggage is often the result of unresolved issues from the past. These issues can include childhood trauma, failed relationships, or unmet needs that continue to affect us in the present. When we don't process and release these emotions, they become stored in our bodies and minds, influencing our behavior, thoughts, and feelings.

Carrying emotional baggage can lead to a range of negative outcomes, including anxiety, depression, and difficulty forming healthy relationships. It can also manifest physically, contributing to stress-related illnesses and chronic pain. Recognizing the impact of emotional baggage is the first step in releasing it.

The Process of Emotional Release

Releasing emotional baggage involves acknowledging and processing the emotions we've been holding onto. This process can be challenging, as it often requires revisiting painful memories and confronting uncomfortable feelings. However, it is a necessary step in the journey of letting go.

One effective approach to emotional release is through therapy or counseling. Working with a trained professional can provide a safe space to explore and process unresolved emotions. Techniques such as cognitive-behavioral therapy (CBT), eye movement desensitization and reprocessing (EMDR), and somatic

experiencing can be particularly
helpful in releasing emotional
baggage.

Another approach is journaling, which
allows you to express your thoughts
and feelings in a structured way.

CHAPTER 4

The Art of Surrender

What It Means to Surrender

The Power of Acceptance

Embracing Uncertainty

Surrender, in the context of personal growth and self-awareness, is often misunderstood. Many perceive surrender as a sign of weakness, a passive resignation to circumstances, or a relinquishment of control. However, true surrender is far from these misconceptions. It is an active, conscious choice to let go of resistance, to accept the present moment as it is, and to trust in the unfolding of life.

To surrender means to release the need to control outcomes, to stop fighting against the flow of life, and to embrace the reality of what is happening right now. This doesn't mean giving up or being passive; rather, it is about finding peace in the present moment, regardless of what that moment holds. It is a powerful act of courage and trust, requiring us to let go of our attachment to how we think things should be and to open ourselves to the possibilities of what could be.

Surrender is often confused with giving up, but the two are fundamentally different. Giving up is an act of defeat, where one relinquishes effort and hope. Surrender, on the other hand, is an act of faith; it is about giving in to the flow of life, trusting that the path ahead, even if uncertain, holds the potential for growth and transformation. In this way, surrender is not an end but a beginning, a doorway to deeper understanding and connection with ourselves and the world around us.

The practice of surrender requires a shift in perspective. Instead of seeing life as something to be controlled and manipulated, we begin to see it as a journey to be experienced, with all its highs and lows. This shift allows us to move from a state of constant striving and tension to one of ease and acceptance. We learn to let go of our rigid expectations and open ourselves to the natural flow of life, trusting that what comes our way is exactly what we need for our growth and evolution.

Surrender also involves letting go of the ego, the part of us that constantly seeks validation, control, and certainty. The ego fears surrender because it equates it with losing power. However, when we surrender, we transcend the ego's limitations and connect with a deeper, more authentic part of ourselves. This deeper self understands that true power comes not from control but from alignment with the flow of life.

In many spiritual traditions, surrender is seen as a path to enlightenment. By letting go of our attachment to outcomes and our desire to control, we align ourselves with a higher power, whether that be the universe, God, or our higher self. This alignment brings a sense of peace and clarity, allowing us to navigate life with greater ease and grace.

The journey of surrender is not always easy. It often requires us to face our fears, to let go of deeply held beliefs and attachments, and to step into the unknown. However, it is through this process of letting go that we find true freedom. We free ourselves from the burden of trying to control the uncontrollable, and we open ourselves to the endless possibilities that life has to offer.

The Power of Acceptance

Acceptance is a fundamental aspect of surrender. To surrender, we must first accept things as they are, without resistance or judgment. Acceptance doesn't mean that we condone or agree with everything that happens, but rather that we acknowledge reality as it is, without trying to change it. This act of acceptance is incredibly powerful, as it frees us from

the suffering that comes from
resisting what is.

When we resist reality, we create
unnecessary stress and tension in
our lives. We expend energy fighting
against what is, rather than using that
energy to move forward and create
positive change. Acceptance allows
us to conserve our energy, to be
present in the moment, and to
respond to life's challenges with
clarity and calmness.

The power of acceptance lies in its
ability to transform our perception of
reality. When we accept things as
they are, we stop seeing ourselves as
victims of circumstance. Instead, we
recognize our ability to choose how
we respond to what happens. This
shift in perception is liberating, as it
empowers us to take responsibility for

our lives and to make conscious, intentional choices.

Acceptance also opens the door to compassion, both for ourselves and others. When we accept our own imperfections and the imperfections of those around us, we become more understanding and less judgmental. We realize that everyone is doing the best they can with the resources they have, and this understanding allows us to approach life with a greater sense of kindness and empathy.

In relationships, acceptance is key to creating deep, meaningful connections. When we accept others as they are, without trying to change them, we create a space for authentic connection. This doesn't mean that we ignore harmful behaviors or accept mistreatment, but rather that we approach relationships with an open heart, recognizing that everyone is on their own unique journey.

Acceptance is also crucial in times of loss or disappointment. When things don't go as planned, or when we experience pain or hardship, it's natural to want to resist or deny what's happening. However, this resistance only prolongs our suffering. By accepting the reality of the situation, we allow ourselves to grieve, to feel the pain, and to eventually heal and move forward.

One of the most profound aspects of acceptance is its ability to bring us peace. When we stop fighting against reality and simply allow ourselves to be present with what is, we experience a deep sense of inner calm. This peace doesn't come from external circumstances but from within, from our ability to be with life as it is, without needing it to be different.

Acceptance is a practice that requires patience and compassion. It's not always easy to accept things as they are, especially when we are faced with challenges or difficulties. However, with practice, we can learn to cultivate acceptance in our lives, and in doing so, we can experience greater peace, freedom, and joy.

Embracing Uncertainty

Uncertainty is an inherent part of life. No matter how much we plan or prepare, we can never fully predict or control what the future holds. This uncertainty can be a source of anxiety and fear, as the unknown often feels threatening and overwhelming. However, when we learn to embrace uncertainty, we

open ourselves to a world of
possibility and potential.

To embrace uncertainty is to
acknowledge that we don't have all
the answers, and that's okay. It's
about letting go of the need to know
and control everything, and instead,
trusting in the process of life. This
trust doesn't come from blind faith but
from a deep understanding that life is
constantly changing and evolving,
and that this change is essential for
growth.

When we embrace uncertainty, we
become more flexible and adaptable.
We learn to go with the flow, to adjust
our sails as the winds of life change
direction. This flexibility allows us to
navigate life's challenges with greater
ease, as we are not rigidly attached
to a specific outcome or plan.
Instead, we are open to the

possibilities that each moment holds, and we trust in our ability to handle whatever comes our way.

Embracing uncertainty also allows us to tap into our creativity and intuition. When we are not fixated on a specific outcome, we are free to explore new ideas, to take risks, and to experiment with different approaches. This openness to the unknown can lead to unexpected discoveries and breakthroughs, as we allow ourselves to think outside the box and to see things from a different perspective.

One of the most powerful aspects of embracing uncertainty is its ability to deepen our connection with ourselves and others. When we are not trying to control or predict the future, we are more present in the moment. This presence allows us to connect with our inner wisdom, to listen to our intuition, and to make decisions that are aligned with our true desires and values.

In relationships, embracing uncertainty allows us to be more authentic and vulnerable. When we let go of the need to know how things will turn out, we are free to be ourselves, to express our true feelings, and to connect with others on a deeper level. This openness and vulnerability can lead to more meaningful and fulfilling relationships, as we are not holding back or trying to protect ourselves from the unknown.

Embracing uncertainty also requires us to confront our fears. The unknown can be scary, as it often brings up feelings of insecurity and doubt. However, by facing these fears head-on, we build resilience and courage. We learn that we can handle whatever comes our way, even if it's not what we expected or wanted.

In many ways, embracing uncertainty is an act of surrender. It's about letting go of our need for control and trusting in the natural flow of life. This doesn't mean that we stop setting goals or making plans, but rather that we approach life with a sense of openness and curiosity, knowing that things may not always go as planned, and that's okay.

The beauty of uncertainty is that it holds the potential for growth and transformation. When we embrace the unknown, we open ourselves to new experiences, new perspectives, and new ways of being. We allow life to surprise us, to take us on unexpected journeys, and to teach us lessons that we might not have learned otherwise.

Ultimately, the art of surrender is a powerful practice that can bring profound peace, freedom, and joy into our lives. By surrendering to the flow of life, accepting things as they are, and embracing uncertainty, we free ourselves from the burden of control and open ourselves to the endless possibilities that life has to offer. This practice requires courage, trust, and patience, but the rewards are well worth the effort. As we learn to surrender, we discover a deeper connection with ourselves and the world around us, and we begin to experience life in a more authentic and meaningful way.

CHAPTER 5

Practical Steps to Letting Go

Decluttering Your Mind and Environment

Mindfulness and Meditation Techniques

Setting Boundaries and Saying No

Decluttering is more than just tidying up; it is an essential practice for creating space in your mind and environment, allowing you to focus on what truly matters. Physical and mental clutter can weigh you down, making it difficult to move forward and embrace change. By addressing both the tangible and intangible aspects of clutter, you can clear a path toward a more peaceful and intentional life.

Understanding the Link Between Physical and Mental Clutter

The relationship between physical and mental clutter is deeply intertwined. A cluttered environment often reflects a cluttered mind, and vice versa. When your surroundings are chaotic, it can lead to feelings of overwhelm, stress, and anxiety. Similarly, when your mind is filled with unresolved thoughts, worries, and distractions, it becomes challenging to maintain a clean and organized space.

To let go of what no longer serves you, it's crucial to address both types of clutter simultaneously. By doing so, you create harmony between your internal and external worlds, paving the way for greater clarity and peace.

Step 1: Decluttering Your Physical Environment

Start Small: The Power of Incremental Progress

Decluttering your physical environment can be a daunting task, especially if you have accumulated a significant amount of belongings over the years. The key to making progress is to start small. Choose a single area to focus on, such as a drawer, a shelf, or a corner of a room. By breaking the task down into manageable chunks, you can avoid feeling overwhelmed and stay motivated as you see tangible results.

The KonMari Method: Keep What Sparks Joy

One popular approach to decluttering is the KonMari Method, developed by Marie Kondo. This method involves sorting through your belongings and only keeping items that "spark joy." While this may sound simple, it requires deep introspection and honesty about what truly adds value to your life. By letting go of items that no longer serve you, you create space for new experiences and opportunities.

The 80/20 Rule: Focusing on the Essentials

The Pareto Principle, or the 80/20 rule, suggests that 80% of the results come from 20% of the effort. Apply this principle to your decluttering process by identifying the 20% of your belongings that you use and love the most. These are the items that should take up the majority of your space. The remaining 80%—which may include items that are rarely used or no longer needed—can be donated, sold, or discarded.

Organizing and Storage Solutions: A Place for Everything

Once you have decluttered, it's important to create an organized system that makes it easy to maintain a clutter-free environment. Invest in storage solutions that work for your space, such as baskets, bins, and shelves. Labeling containers and designating specific spots for items will help ensure that everything has a place and can be easily found when needed.

Maintaining a Clutter-Free Space: Daily Habits for Success

Decluttering is not a one-time event but an ongoing process. To maintain a clutter-free environment, develop daily habits that prevent clutter from accumulating. Simple practices such as tidying up before bed, putting items back in their designated spots, and regularly reassessing your belongings can help keep your space organized and peaceful.

Step 2: Decluttering Your Mind

Mindfulness: Bringing Awareness to Your Thoughts

Just as physical clutter can accumulate in your environment, mental clutter can build up in your mind. One effective way to declutter your mind is through mindfulness—a practice that involves bringing your full attention to the present moment without judgment. By observing your thoughts as they arise, you can begin to recognize patterns and let go of those that no longer serve you.

Journaling: Unloading Your Thoughts on Pamper

Journaling is a powerful tool for decluttering your mind. When you write down your thoughts, feelings, and worries, you externalize them, making it easier to process and release them. Journaling can also help you gain clarity on issues that may be causing mental clutter, allowing you to address them more effectively.

Prioritization: Focusing on What Truly Matters

Mental clutter often stems from trying to juggle too many tasks and responsibilities at once. To declutter your mind, prioritize your to-do list by focusing on what truly matters. Identify the most important tasks that align with your goals and values, and let go of or delegate the rest. By narrowing your focus, you reduce mental overload and increase your productivity.

Meditation: Creating Space for Stillness

Meditation is another powerful practice for decluttering your mind. By setting aside time each day to sit in stillness, you create space for mental clarity and peace. Meditation helps you detach from the constant stream of thoughts and worries, allowing you to observe them from a distance rather than becoming entangled in them.

Limiting Information Overload: Managing Digital Clutter

In today's digital age, information overload is a common source of mental clutter. Constant notifications, emails, and social media updates can overwhelm your mind, making it difficult to focus. To declutter your mind, take steps to manage digital clutter. This might involve setting boundaries for screen time, unsubscribing from unnecessary emails, and organizing your digital files. By reducing the amount of information you consume, you create more mental space for what truly matters.

Step 3: The Emotional Aspect of Decluttering

Letting Go of Sentimental Items: Navigating Emotional Attachments

One of the most challenging aspects of decluttering is letting go of sentimental items—those belongings that hold emotional significance. While these items may evoke memories and emotions, holding onto too many can weigh you down. To navigate this process, consider whether the item truly adds value to your life or if it's the memory attached to it that you cherish. If it's the latter, consider alternative ways to honor the memory, such as taking a photo of the item or creating a scrapbook.

Forgiveness: Releasing Emotional Clutter

Emotional clutter often takes the form of unresolved feelings, grudges, and regrets. Holding onto these emotions can cloud your mind and prevent you from moving forward. One of the most powerful ways to declutter emotionally is through forgiveness—both of others and yourself. By letting go of past hurts and mistakes, you free yourself from the burden of carrying them with you.

Gratitude: Shifting Focus to the Positive

Gratitude is a powerful antidote to emotional clutter. When you focus on what you're grateful for, you shift your attention away from what's lacking or causing distress. Practicing gratitude regularly can help you maintain a positive mindset and reduce the impact of negative emotions on your mental and emotional well-being.

Step 4: Creating and Maintaining Boundaries

Setting Boundaries in Your Environment

A crucial step in maintaining a clutter-free environment is setting boundaries—both physical and mental. In your physical space, this might involve establishing rules for what comes into your home and where it goes. For example, you might decide that new items must replace something old or that certain areas of your home should remain clutter-free zones.

Setting Boundaries in Your Mind

Just as physical boundaries are important, so too are mental boundaries. These involve protecting your mental space from negative influences and unnecessary distractions. This might include setting limits on how much time you spend on social media, saying no to commitments that don't align with your priorities, and practicing self-care to recharge your mental energy.

Enforcing Boundaries: The Importance of Consistency

Once you've set boundaries, it's important to enforce them consistently. This requires discipline and self-awareness. When you notice that clutter—whether physical or mental—is starting to accumulate, take action immediately to address it. Consistent enforcement of boundaries will help you maintain the progress you've made and prevent future clutter from taking over.

Step 5: The Long-Term Benefits of Decluttering

Improved Mental Clarity and Focus

One of the most immediate benefits of decluttering your mind and environment is improved mental clarity and focus. When you remove unnecessary distractions and create a clean, organized space, your mind is better able to concentrate on the tasks at hand. This increased focus can lead to greater productivity, creativity, and overall well-being.

Enhanced Emotional Well-Being

Decluttering also has a profound impact on your emotional well-being. By letting go of physical items and mental burdens that no longer serve you, you create space for positive emotions and experiences. This can lead to a greater sense of peace, contentment, and emotional resilience.

Increased Energy and Motivation

Clutter—whether physical or mental—can drain your energy and motivation. When your environment is chaotic or your mind is cluttered, it's easy to feel overwhelmed and stuck.

By decluttering, you remove these obstacles, freeing up energy that can be redirected toward more fulfilling activities and goals.

Greater Alignment with Your Values and Goals

Decluttering helps you align your environment and mindset with your values and goals. When you let go of what no longer serves you, you create space for what truly matters. This alignment can lead to a more intentional and purposeful life, where your surroundings and thoughts support your aspirations.

What is Mindfulness?

Mindfulness is the practice of being fully present in the moment without judgment. It involves paying attention to your thoughts, feelings, and physical sensations, allowing you to observe them with curiosity and compassion. Mindfulness doesn't mean eliminating thoughts or emotions but rather noticing them as they arise and letting them pass without becoming attached or overwhelmed.

One of the most powerful aspects of mindfulness is its ability to anchor you in the here and now. Often, our minds are caught up in the past or future—regretting what has happened or worrying about what might occur. Mindfulness teaches you to focus on what is happening right now, helping to quiet mental chatter and reduce anxiety.

Benefits of Mindfulness

The benefits of mindfulness are vast, ranging from psychological to physiological:

1. Reduced Stress and Anxiety: Mindfulness helps regulate emotions, making it easier to manage stress and reduce anxiety. By focusing on the present, you're less likely to ruminate on past events or worry about the future.

2. Improved Focus and Concentration: Mindfulness trains the mind to stay present, which improves concentration and enhances productivity.

3. Better Emotional Regulation: Mindfulness enables you to be more aware of your emotions, helping you

respond to situations with clarity and calm rather than reacting impulsively.

4. Increased Self-Awareness: Through mindfulness, you develop a deeper understanding of your thoughts and behaviors, fostering personal growth and emotional intelligence.

5. Improved Physical Health: Studies have shown that mindfulness can improve immune function, lower blood pressure, and reduce symptoms of chronic pain.

Mindfulness Practices

Incorporating mindfulness into your life doesn't require a complete overhaul of your routine. There are several simple practices you can adopt, even amidst a busy schedule.

1. Mindful Breathing: One of the easiest ways to practice mindfulness is to focus on your breath. Take a few minutes each day to pay attention to the sensation of breathing in and out. Notice the rise and fall of your chest and how the air feels as it enters and leaves your nostrils. This practice helps center your mind and bring you back to the present.

2. Body Scan: A body scan involves bringing awareness to different parts of your body, noticing any tension, discomfort, or sensations. Start at your toes and work your way up to your head, observing how each part of your body feels without judgment. This technique helps you reconnect with your physical self and relax.

3. Mindful Eating: Eating can become an automatic activity where you're distracted by thoughts, devices, or external stimuli. Mindful eating encourages you to savor each bite, paying attention to the texture, flavor, and aroma of your food. This practice can foster a healthier relationship with food and promote better digestion.

4. Mindful Walking: Whether you're walking to work or taking a stroll in nature, mindful walking involves paying attention to the sensation of your feet touching the ground, the rhythm of your steps, and the sights and sounds around you. This simple practice helps cultivate mindfulness while staying active.

5. Mindfulness in Daily Activities: Everyday tasks like washing dishes or brushing your teeth can become mindful moments. Focus on the

sensory experience of the task—how the water feels, the sound of the brush, or the smell of soap. These small practices can transform mundane activities into opportunities for mindfulness.

What is Meditation?

Meditation is a formal practice that involves training the mind to focus and achieve a heightened state of awareness. Unlike mindfulness, which can be practiced throughout daily activities, meditation often involves setting aside time for stillness and reflection. There are many types of meditation, but they all share the goal of calming the mind and deepening self-awareness.

Benefits of Meditation

Meditation has been practiced for thousands of years, and its benefits are well-documented:

1. Stress Reduction: Meditation helps calm the mind and body, lowering stress levels by promoting relaxation and reducing cortisol, the body's stress hormone.

2. Enhanced Focus and Clarity: By regularly meditating, you train your mind to focus better, which improves cognitive function and clarity of thought.

3. Better Emotional Health: Meditation has been shown to reduce symptoms of depression and anxiety while improving overall mood and emotional resilience.

4. Physical Health Improvements: Regular meditation can improve sleep, lower blood pressure, and enhance immune function.

Meditation Techniques

There are many different meditation techniques to choose from, depending on your goals and preferences:

1. Focused Attention Meditation: This involves focusing on a single point, such as your breath, a candle flame, or a mantra. Whenever your mind wanders, gently bring it back to the object of focus. This practice helps improve concentration and calm the mind.

2. Loving-Kindness Meditation: Also known as Metta meditation, this

practice involves generating feelings of love and compassion for yourself and others. You repeat phrases like "May I be happy, may I be healthy, may I be safe" and gradually extend these wishes to others. This meditation fosters empathy, kindness, and emotional healing.

3. Body Scan Meditation: Similar to the mindfulness body scan, this meditation involves systematically focusing on different parts of your body, promoting relaxation and physical awareness.

4. Guided Meditation: In guided meditation, a teacher or recording leads you through the practice, often incorporating visualization or storytelling. This is a great option for beginners or those looking for specific guidance.

5. Transcendental Meditation: This technique involves silently repeating a mantra to settle the mind into a state of restful awareness. It's often practiced for 20 minutes twice a day and has been shown to reduce stress and improve mental clarity.

Setting Boundaries and Saying No

In today's society, the ability to set boundaries and say no is essential for maintaining mental and emotional well-being. Without healthy boundaries, you risk feeling overwhelmed, drained, and resentful. Saying no is not about rejecting others but about protecting your own space, time, and energy.

The Importance of Setting Boundaries

Boundaries are the limits we set to protect our physical, emotional, and mental well-being. They define where your needs and priorities begin and where others' expectations and demands end. Setting boundaries is crucial for maintaining healthy relationships, reducing stress, and preserving your sense of self.

Benefits of Healthy Boundaries

1. Improved Relationships: Healthy boundaries foster respect and understanding in relationships. When others know your limits, they are more likely to honor them, creating a balanced dynamic.

2. Reduced Stress and Burnout: By setting boundaries, you prevent yourself from becoming overcommitted or taking on more than you can handle, reducing the risk of burnout.

3. Increased Self-Esteem: Setting boundaries is a form of self-respect. It shows that you value your needs and are willing to prioritize them, boosting your confidence and sense of worth.

4. Better Emotional Health: Boundaries protect you from emotional harm by preventing others from encroaching on your personal space or taking advantage of your kindness.

Common Types of Boundaries

1. Physical Boundaries: These involve your personal space, privacy, and body. You have the right to decide how much physical contact you're comfortable with and who is allowed into your personal space.

2. Emotional Boundaries: Emotional boundaries protect your feelings and emotional well-being. They involve setting limits on how much emotional energy you give to others and deciding how you want to be treated in emotional situations.

3. Time Boundaries: Time boundaries protect your schedule and time. They involve saying no to commitments that don't align with your priorities or that would overwhelm your schedule.

4. Mental Boundaries: Mental boundaries protect your thoughts and beliefs. You have the right to hold your own opinions and beliefs without being pressured to conform to others.

5. Material Boundaries: Material boundaries involve your possessions and finances. They protect your right

to decide how your belongings or money are used.

How to Set Boundaries

Setting boundaries may feel uncomfortable at first, especially if you're used to saying yes to everyone. However, with practice, it becomes easier and more empowering.

1. Identify Your Limits: The first step in setting boundaries is understanding your limits. Reflect on situations where you've felt uncomfortable, stressed, or overwhelmed. These are likely areas where you need to set boundaries.

2. Communicate Clearly: When setting boundaries, be clear and direct. Use "I" statements to express your needs and avoid blaming or accusing others. For example, say, "I

need some time to myself" rather than "You're always demanding my time."

3. Be Consistent: Once you've set a boundary, it's important to stick to it. Inconsistency can confuse others and lead to boundary violations. If someone crosses a boundary, calmly remind them of your limit.

4. Practice Self-Care: Setting boundaries is an act of self-care. It's about protecting your well-being and ensuring that you have the time and energy to care for yourself. Remember, you don't need to feel guilty for putting yourself first.

5. Be Prepared for Pushback: Not everyone will respond positively to your boundaries, especially if they've benefited from you not having them in the past. Stay firm and remember that

setting boundaries is about protecting
your peace.

CHAPTER 6

Transforming Pain into Growth

Healing Past Wounds

Turning Loss into Strength

Finding Purpose in Pain

Pain is an inevitable part of life. It manifests in different forms—physical, emotional, mental—and challenges us in ways we often feel unprepared to handle. However, pain doesn't have to be purely destructive. Through mindful engagement with our struggles, we can transform pain into growth, evolving into stronger, wiser individuals. This process, while difficult, is deeply empowering and provides the foundation for resilience, strength, and purpose. In this section, we'll explore the path of transforming pain by addressing past wounds, turning loss into strength, and finding meaning in suffering.

Healing Past Wounds

The pain of our past can cling to us like an invisible weight, affecting our decisions, relationships, and worldview. Past wounds—whether emotional, psychological, or physical—can keep us stuck in cycles of suffering if left unaddressed. Healing is not an overnight process; it requires patience, intention, and, most importantly, the willingness to confront what hurts. The journey of healing past wounds can be broken down into several steps:

Acknowledging the Pain

The first step toward healing is acknowledging the existence of pain. Too often, people bury their pain in an attempt to move on or appear strong, but unresolved pain festers and manifests in unhealthy behaviors, such as anger, anxiety, depression, or self-sabotage. It's important to create a safe space to feel and express these emotions. Journaling, therapy, and honest conversations with trusted friends or loved ones can help bring buried emotions to the surface.

Acknowledging pain doesn't mean becoming consumed by it. It's about accepting that it's part of the human experience and that feeling it is the first step toward recovery. Denying or suppressing pain only prolongs the healing process and can intensify its impact over time.

Forgiveness as a Tool for Healing

One of the most difficult yet vital aspects of healing is forgiveness. This doesn't mean excusing harmful behavior or invalidating the pain you've experienced. Rather, it involves releasing the hold that the person or event has over your emotions. Holding on to anger or resentment keeps you trapped in a cycle of suffering. Forgiveness allows you to reclaim your emotional freedom and shift your focus toward growth and healing.

Forgiveness also includes forgiving yourself. Many people carry guilt or shame for their past actions or for allowing themselves to stay in painful situations. Self-forgiveness is essential to healing because it removes the burden of self-condemnation, allowing space for self-compassion and acceptance.

Rewriting the Narrative

Past wounds often shape the way we see ourselves and the world. Healing involves rewriting the narrative of those wounds. Instead of viewing yourself as a victim of your circumstances, you can choose to see yourself as a survivor or even a thriver. Rewriting your story isn't about denying what happened but about reclaiming your power in the face of adversity.

For example, someone who experienced childhood neglect may have spent years believing they are unworthy of love. In healing, they can recognize that their worth was never defined by the actions of others. They can start to see their resilience, strength, and ability to give and receive love despite their past experiences.

Embracing Vulnerability

Vulnerability is often seen as a weakness, but in the context of healing, it's a tremendous strength. When you allow yourself to be vulnerable, you open yourself to healing on a deeper level. Vulnerability means admitting that you're hurting, that you need help, and that you're willing to face your pain in order to heal.

Healing doesn't happen in isolation. Connecting with others and sharing your pain, whether through therapy, support groups, or close relationships, fosters a sense of community and understanding. It allows you to release bottled-up emotions and receive the support needed to heal.

Turning Loss into Strength

Loss, whether it's the death of a loved one, the end of a relationship, or the loss of a job or opportunity, is one of the most painful experiences we endure as humans. However, loss can also be a profound teacher, offering us the opportunity to grow in ways we never imagined. By shifting our perspective on loss, we can transform it into a source of strength and resilience.

Accepting the Reality of Loss

The first step in transforming loss into strength is accepting the reality of what has been lost. Denial, while a common coping mechanism, prevents us from fully processing the loss. It's only through acceptance that we can begin to grieve and, eventually, heal.

Acceptance doesn't mean that we no longer feel pain. Instead, it means recognizing that pain is a natural response to loss and allowing ourselves to feel it without resistance. Grieving is a necessary process for healing, and everyone moves through it in their own time. By honoring our grief, we create space for healing and growth.

Finding Meaning in Loss

One of the ways we can transform loss into strength is by finding meaning in the experience. This doesn't mean that the loss itself was necessary or justified, but that we can extract valuable lessons from it. For instance, the loss of a relationship may teach us more about our emotional needs and boundaries, while the loss of a loved one may deepen our appreciation for life and the time we have with others.

Many people who experience profound loss find themselves reevaluating their priorities and values. This reevaluation often leads to a greater sense of purpose and clarity in life. While the loss itself is painful, the growth that comes from it can lead to a richer, more meaningful existence.

Building Resilience Through Loss

Loss forces us to confront our vulnerability and the impermanence of life. This realization can be both terrifying and liberating. By accepting that nothing in life is guaranteed or permanent, we build resilience—the ability to adapt and bounce back from difficult situations.

Resilience doesn't mean that we no longer feel pain; it means that we learn to navigate through it with strength and grace. Each time we face loss and emerge on the other side, we strengthen our ability to handle future challenges. Over time, we develop a deeper sense of trust in ourselves and our capacity to overcome adversity.

Channeling Pain into Purpose

One of the most powerful ways to transform loss into strength is by channeling our pain into a greater purpose. Many people who experience profound loss go on to create something meaningful from their pain—whether it's starting a nonprofit, writing a book, or dedicating their lives to helping others facing similar struggles.

By using our pain as a catalyst for positive change, we give our suffering meaning and turn it into something that serves others. This shift from focusing on our own pain to helping others is often the key to healing and growth.

Finding Purpose in Pain

Pain, when approached mindfully, can be a doorway to profound personal growth and transformation. Rather than seeing pain as an enemy, we can begin to view it as a teacher—a guide that helps us uncover deeper truths about ourselves and the world. Finding purpose in pain allows us to transcend suffering and use it as a tool for growth.

Pain as a Teacher

Every painful experience has something to teach us. Pain forces us to slow down, reflect, and reevaluate our lives. It calls our attention to areas that need healing, change, or growth. For instance, emotional pain may indicate unresolved trauma or unaddressed emotional needs, while physical pain may signal that our bodies need care and attention.

By viewing pain as a teacher rather than a punishment, we open ourselves to the lessons it has to offer. This shift in perspective allows us to approach pain with curiosity and openness rather than fear and avoidance.

Discovering Inner Strength

One of the most powerful outcomes of finding purpose in pain is the discovery of our inner strength. Pain often forces us to dig deep within ourselves, revealing reserves of strength and resilience we didn't know we had. It's through facing and overcoming pain that we realize just how strong and capable we are.

The experience of enduring and overcoming pain builds confidence in our ability to handle life's challenges. It teaches us that we are not defined by our circumstances but by how we respond to them. This realization can be incredibly empowering and serves as a foundation for future growth.

Cultivating Empathy and Compassion

Experiencing pain, especially deep emotional pain, often makes us more empathetic and compassionate toward others. When we've been through suffering, we are more likely to understand and relate to the pain of others. This empathy can lead to deeper connections with those around us and a greater desire to help and support others in their struggles.

In this way, pain can be a source of connection and community. It reminds us that suffering is a universal experience and that we are not alone in our struggles. This shared understanding fosters compassion and encourages us to show kindness, not only to others but also to ourselves.

Reframing Suffering as Growth

While pain is often viewed as something to be avoided or eliminated, reframing it as an opportunity for growth allows us to approach it with a new mindset. Instead of asking, "Why is this happening to me?" we can ask, "What can I learn from this?" This shift in perspective transforms pain from a source of suffering into a catalyst for personal and spiritual growth.

Reframing suffering doesn't mean that we dismiss or minimize the pain we feel. It means that we recognize its potential to lead us to greater wisdom, strength, and understanding. By embracing pain as part of our journey, we open ourselves to the possibility of transformation.

In other words embracing the Transformational Power of Pain

Pain is an inevitable part of the human experience, but it doesn't have to define or defeat us. By engaging with our pain mindfully and with intention, we can transform it into a source of growth and strength. Healing past wounds, turning loss into strength, and finding purpose in pain allows us to emerge from suffering as stronger, more resilient individuals.

The process of transforming pain into growth is not linear or easy. It requires patience, self-compassion, and a willingness to face difficult emotions.

CHAPTER 7

Embracing Forgiveness

Forgiving Yourself and Others

The Freedom of Letting Go of Grudges

Moving Forward with Compassion

Forgiveness is often described as a powerful, transformative experience, but for many, it remains elusive. We may be conditioned to believe that forgiving others—and even more so, forgiving ourselves—is an impossible or unnecessary task. In reality, forgiveness is an essential part of healing, growth, and personal freedom. Without it, we remain tethered to the past, carrying the weight of resentment, guilt, and shame. This section will explore the dual nature of forgiveness: forgiving others and forgiving oneself. By understanding and embracing forgiveness, we can break free from emotional burdens and move forward with peace and grace.

The Nature of Forgiveness

To embrace forgiveness, it's essential to first understand what it is and what it is not. Forgiveness is not about condoning wrongdoing, excusing harm, or pretending that hurtful actions never occurred. Instead, it is a conscious decision to let go of the pain and bitterness that keep us emotionally shackled to the past.

When we forgive, we do not erase the past or diminish the significance of what happened. Rather, we release the power it has over us. We choose to rise above the feelings of anger and resentment, allowing ourselves to heal. Forgiveness is a gift we give ourselves, one that liberates us from emotional bondage and creates space for love, peace, and personal growth.

In this sense, forgiveness is less about the other person and more about our own emotional well-being. Whether it's forgiving someone who hurt us or forgiving ourselves for mistakes we've made, the goal is to free our hearts and minds from the negativity that impedes our progress.

Why Forgiveness Matters

The act of forgiveness has profound psychological, emotional, and even physical benefits. Research shows that forgiveness can reduce stress, anxiety, and depression, while improving self-esteem, relationships, and overall well-being. People who are able to forgive tend to have lower blood pressure, a stronger immune system, and a greater sense of life satisfaction.

But beyond the physical and psychological benefits, forgiveness is a spiritual practice that aligns us with higher truths. In many religious and philosophical traditions, forgiveness is seen as a divine attribute, a reflection of love, compassion, and grace. By forgiving others and ourselves, we align with these higher principles, creating a deeper connection to our own inner wisdom and spiritual path.

Forgiving Others

Forgiving others can be one of the most challenging acts of compassion we undertake. When we are wronged, our natural inclination is to protect ourselves from further harm, often by holding onto anger, resentment, or a desire for revenge. In some cases, we may even feel justified in harboring these negative emotions, especially if the offense was severe.

However, refusing to forgive only deepens our wounds and prolongs our suffering. It creates an emotional prison where we replay the hurt over and over in our minds, reliving the pain without finding resolution. To forgive others is to acknowledge the harm they've caused while choosing to release the grip it has on our hearts. It's not about reconciliation or restoring trust; rather, it's about freeing ourselves from the toxicity of resentment.

Steps to Forgiving Others

1. Acknowledge the Hurt

Forgiveness begins with an honest acknowledgment of the hurt we've experienced. Denying or minimizing the pain does not help in the healing process. We must allow ourselves to fully feel and understand the impact of the wrongdoing, no matter how difficult it may be. It's important to validate our emotions rather than suppress them.

2. Empathize with the Offender

While it may seem counterintuitive, empathy is a powerful tool in the forgiveness process. Empathy does not mean excusing harmful behavior, but rather recognizing that the person who hurt us is flawed, just like we are. People act out of their own pain, confusion, and unresolved issues. Understanding this can help us shift from anger to compassion.

3. Let Go of the Desire for Revenge

When we hold onto a desire for revenge, we perpetuate the cycle of pain. Instead of seeking retribution, we can choose to let go. This doesn't mean that we ignore justice, but we release our need to personally punish the offender. By relinquishing this need, we reclaim our power and start the journey toward healing.

4. Decide to Forgive

Forgiveness is a conscious choice. It may not happen overnight, and it certainly does not require us to feel "ready." But at some point, we must decide that holding onto the hurt is no longer serving us. This decision marks the beginning of a new chapter, one where we are no longer defined by the pain of the past.

5. Release and Move On

Once we've made the decision to forgive, the final step is to release the emotional burden and move forward. This doesn't mean forgetting or pretending the hurt never happened. Instead, we let go of the emotional charge that the event holds over us. We accept that the past cannot be changed, and we focus on creating a future that is free from the weight of resentment.

Forgiving Yourself

While forgiving others can be difficult, forgiving ourselves is often an even greater challenge. We are often our own harshest critics, replaying our mistakes and shortcomings in our minds, convinced that we do not deserve forgiveness. Self-forgiveness requires us to confront our own guilt, shame, and self-judgment with compassion and understanding.

The inability to forgive ourselves can manifest in various ways—constant self-blame, feelings of unworthiness, and a deep-seated sense of guilt that prevents us from moving forward. These feelings can stem from past mistakes, failures, or times when we believe we've let ourselves or others down. However, just as we would extend compassion to others, we must learn to offer it to ourselves.

The Importance of Self-Forgiveness

When we refuse to forgive ourselves, we remain stuck in the past, unable to fully embrace the present or the future. Self-forgiveness is not about denying responsibility for our actions, but rather accepting our humanity and recognizing that we are all works in progress. Everyone makes mistakes, and these mistakes do not define our worth.

By practicing self-forgiveness, we release the burden of guilt and shame, creating space for self-love, healing, and personal growth. We allow ourselves to learn from our past, rather than being imprisoned by it. In doing so, we reclaim our power and our right to move forward with a sense of peace and purpose.

Steps to Forgiving Yourself

1. Acknowledge Your Mistakes

Just as with forgiving others, the first step in self-forgiveness is acknowledging the mistakes or wrongdoings that are causing you guilt or shame. It's important to face these feelings head-on, rather than avoiding or suppressing them. By confronting the emotions associated with your past actions, you take the first step toward healing.

2. Understand the Impact

Take time to reflect on the impact of your actions, both on yourself and on others. This self-reflection is not about self-punishment, but about gaining clarity and understanding. By understanding the consequences of your actions, you can take responsibility for them in a healthy way, without being overwhelmed by guilt.

3. Practice Self-Compassion

Self-compassion is the cornerstone of self-forgiveness. It involves treating yourself with the same kindness, understanding, and empathy that you would offer to a loved one. Recognize that you are human, and like all humans, you are imperfect. You are allowed to make mistakes, and you are allowed to learn and grow from them.

4. Learn from the Experience

Every mistake offers an opportunity for growth and learning. Instead of dwelling on the guilt and shame, ask yourself what lessons you can take from the experience. How can you use this knowledge to improve yourself and make better choices in the future? By reframing your mistakes as learning opportunities, you transform them into stepping stones toward personal development.

5. Release the Guilt

Once you've acknowledged your mistakes, taken responsibility, and learned from the experience, it's time to release the guilt and shame. Holding onto these emotions only keeps you stuck in the past. Let go of the self-blame and allow yourself to move forward with a sense of peace and acceptance. You deserve forgiveness, just as much as anyone else.

The Intersection of Forgiving Yourself and Others

Often, forgiving ourselves and forgiving others are interconnected. When we hold grudges against others, we may also be harboring feelings of guilt or shame about our own role in the situation. Conversely, when we struggle to forgive ourselves, it can be difficult to extend forgiveness to others. By embracing both self-forgiveness and the forgiveness of others, we create a holistic path to healing.

The Freedom of Forgiveness

Forgiveness is a powerful act of liberation. Whether we are forgiving others or forgiving ourselves, the process allows us to release the emotional burdens that keep us tied to the past. Through forgiveness, we reclaim our power, heal our hearts, and create space for peace, love, and growth. It is not always an easy journey, but it is one that ultimately leads to freedom and transformation.

Embracing forgiveness requires courage, compassion, and a

willingness to let go. It is a profound act of self-love, one that not only heals old wounds but also opens the door to a brighter, more fulfilling future. By forgiving others and ourselves, we free our spirits from the weight of resentment, guilt, and shame, allowing us to live with greater joy, grace, and inner peace.

The Freedom of Letting Go of Grudges

Grudges are often rooted in a perceived injustice or betrayal, and holding onto them can feel like a form of protection. When we harbor resentment toward someone, it may seem like we're keeping a barrier between ourselves and future hurt. However, this barrier often serves as a prison, locking us in a cycle of anger, pain, and bitterness.

The emotional weight of a grudge is heavy. It can manifest in various forms: anxiety, sleeplessness, and even physical ailments. Psychologically, holding onto a grudge keeps us tethered to the very event that caused the pain, continuously reliving it in our minds. This creates a loop where the pain is refreshed, rather than allowed to fade. We may believe that by holding on, we are somehow punishing the person who wronged us, but in reality, we are only harming ourselves.

The energy spent maintaining a grudge is substantial. Anger and resentment require constant emotional fuel, which can drain our mental resources. This constant replaying of the hurt stifles our capacity for joy and keeps us from living fully in the present moment.

The Illusion of Control

Grudges give us an illusion of control. We may believe that by not forgiving, we hold some power over the person who wronged us. We might convince ourselves that forgiving them would somehow minimize the wrong they committed or make us vulnerable again. Yet, the control we think we are exercising is an illusion. In reality, the grudge controls us, dictating our thoughts and behaviors, and often causing us to act in ways we otherwise would not.

Letting go of a grudge is not about relinquishing control but about reclaiming it. When we hold onto grudges, we allow the person or situation that hurt us to dictate our emotional state. By letting go, we take back that power. Forgiveness becomes an act of self-empowerment, where we choose not to let the past dominate our present.

The Physical and Emotional Toll

The link between grudges and physical health is well documented. Holding onto anger and resentment can trigger the body's stress response, leading to increased blood pressure, tension, and even a compromised immune system. Over time, this can result in chronic conditions such as heart disease and high blood pressure.

Emotionally, grudges cloud our relationships. They prevent us from fully connecting with others because we are often guarded, afraid of experiencing the same hurt again. This can lead to feelings of isolation and loneliness, even when surrounded by loved ones. The pain of the past begins to color our interactions with others, often leading to misunderstandings and conflicts.

Letting go of a grudge allows us to release these toxic emotions and their corresponding physical effects. It gives us the freedom to be fully present with others, unburdened by the emotional baggage of the past.

The Path to Freedom

True freedom comes when we make the conscious decision to release the grudge. This process often involves a deep level of self-reflection and emotional work. It requires us to confront the pain we have been holding onto and examine the root causes of our resentment. Often, this means acknowledging our own vulnerabilities, fears, and unmet expectations.

Forgiveness does not mean condoning the behavior or forgetting the harm done. Instead, it is about releasing the emotional hold that the event or person has over us. This is a personal journey, one that requires patience and compassion toward ourselves. The freedom that comes from letting go of a grudge is not just about the absence of anger, but the presence of peace.

The process of letting go is deeply personal and may take time. However, the more we practice it, the more we begin to experience a lightness in our being. This lightness allows us to approach life with greater openness, enabling us to experience more joy, love, and connection.

Moving Forward with Compassion

Understanding Compassion

Compassion is a powerful antidote to the bitterness that grudges create. It is the ability to understand and empathize with the pain of others, even those who have hurt us. Moving forward with compassion does not mean accepting wrongdoing or inviting more harm into our lives, but rather, recognizing the humanity in others, even in their imperfections and mistakes.

When we cultivate compassion, we allow ourselves to see beyond the hurt and into the broader picture of human experience. People act out of their own wounds, fears, and ignorance, and while this does not excuse harmful behavior, it does help us understand it. Compassion shifts our focus from seeking retribution to seeking understanding, from punishment to healing.

Compassion for Ourselves

Before we can extend compassion to others, we must first extend it to ourselves. Self-compassion is a critical aspect of healing and letting go of grudges. When we are hurt, it's easy to fall into self-blame, questioning why we allowed ourselves to be in a vulnerable position. We may replay the event, wondering what we could have done differently. This self-critical thinking only deepens our pain.

Self-compassion means accepting that we are human, that we will experience pain, and that we are deserving of love and understanding even in our weakest moments. It allows us to acknowledge our hurt without judgment, offering ourselves the same kindness we would offer a close friend.

As we begin to heal through self-compassion, we build the emotional strength needed to forgive others. The act of forgiving becomes less about excusing the harm and more about releasing ourselves from the emotional burden of the grudge.

Compassion for Others

Forgiving others is a profound act of compassion. It allows us to acknowledge their humanity, their fallibility, and their capacity for growth and change. In choosing compassion, we open the door to seeing the person who wronged us as someone who, like us, is on their own journey of healing and self-discovery.

Compassion doesn't mean that we must maintain relationships with those who have hurt us, nor does it mean that we have to accept their behavior. What it does mean is that we choose not to let their actions define us or dictate our future. It's a conscious decision to let go of the desire for revenge or retribution and instead focus on our own growth and healing.

When we move forward with compassion, we shift our energy from the past to the present. We begin to focus on how we can live more fully, love more openly, and connect more deeply with others.

The Ripple Effect of Compassion

When we choose compassion, the effects extend far beyond ourselves. Compassion has a ripple effect, positively influencing those around us. When we forgive and release grudges, we model for others what it means to live with grace and empathy. This can inspire those in our circle to adopt similar attitudes, fostering an environment of mutual respect and kindness.

In relationships, compassion can mend what was once broken. It paves the way for open communication, understanding, and reconciliation. Even if reconciliation is not possible, compassion allows us to let go of the anger and resentment that might otherwise consume us.

The power of compassion lies in its ability to transform not just our inner world, but also the world around us.

By moving forward with compassion, we contribute to a culture of understanding, where forgiveness and healing become more attainable for all.

Living a Life of Compassion

Moving forward with compassion is not a one-time act but a way of life. It involves a commitment to seeing the world and others through the lens of empathy and kindness. This does not mean that we will never feel anger or hurt again, but that when these emotions arise, we respond to them with awareness and understanding rather than with bitterness and blame.

Living a compassionate life means making choices that align with our values of empathy, understanding, and forgiveness. It means creating boundaries that protect our well-being while still maintaining an open heart toward others. It means recognizing that compassion is a strength, not a weakness, and that by extending it to others, we are also healing ourselves.

In our daily interactions, choosing compassion can manifest in small yet meaningful ways. Whether it's offering a kind word to a stranger, listening without judgment to a friend, or extending forgiveness to someone who has wronged us, these acts create a ripple of positivity that can have a profound impact.

Therefore, it's clear that the freedom that comes from letting go of grudges and moving forward with compassion is profound. It frees us from the emotional chains that keep us bound to the past, allowing us to live more fully in the present. By releasing grudges, we reclaim our power, and by choosing compassion, we create a life filled with love, peace, and understanding.

This freedom is not only a gift we give to ourselves but also to those around us. It allows us to contribute to a world where forgiveness and compassion are valued, where healing is possible, and where we can all move forward with a greater sense of peace and connection.

As we practice letting go and embracing compassion, we begin to experience life more fully, with an open heart and a clear mind. We are no longer burdened by the weight of the past, and we can step into a future where forgiveness and compassion guide our way.

CHAPTER 8

Creating Space for New Opportunities

The Law of Attraction and Letting Go

Inviting Abundance and Joy

Cultivating a Growth Mindset

Opportunities often present themselves when we make room for them in our lives. When we cling to old habits, outdated beliefs, or environments that no longer serve us, we unintentionally block the path to new possibilities. Letting go of what weighs us down allows for fresh energy to flow into our lives, creating the space needed for growth, abundance, and joy.

The Law of Attraction and Letting Go

The Law of Attraction is rooted in the belief that like attracts like—what we focus on expands, and our thoughts, feelings, and beliefs directly shape the reality we experience. If our minds and lives are cluttered with negativity, fear, or attachment to things that no longer serve us, we limit the energy available to attract new and positive experiences. Letting go is a crucial component of harnessing the Law of Attraction because it allows us to make space for what we truly desire.

Releasing Limiting Beliefs

One of the biggest blocks to attracting what we want is our own set of limiting beliefs. These are often deeply ingrained ideas about ourselves and the world that dictate what we believe is possible. These beliefs might sound like:

- "I'm not good enough to achieve that goal."

- "Success is for other people, not me."

- "Things never work out for me."

When we hold onto these limiting thoughts, we send out the vibration of lack and inadequacy into the universe. As a result, the Law of Attraction will reflect that energy back to us in the form of missed opportunities, frustration, or continued stagnation. To create space for new opportunities, we must identify and release these limiting beliefs.

Letting go of these beliefs involves an active process of self-awareness and reframing. One powerful tool is cognitive restructuring, where we challenge these negative beliefs and replace them with affirmations that align with our desires:

- "I am capable and deserving of success."

- "Abundance is always flowing toward me."

- "I trust the process and know things are working in my favor."

Emotional Release and Energy Shifts

In addition to our thoughts, our emotions play a critical role in the

Law of Attraction. Holding onto negative emotions like resentment, anger, or fear can block the flow of positive energy. Letting go of these emotions is vital for creating space for new opportunities.

Emotional release can take many forms, from journaling about past grievances to practicing forgiveness toward those who have wronged us, or even simply acknowledging and processing emotions in a healthy way. Once these emotions are released, our energy shifts from contraction to expansion, opening us up to attract positive experiences.

Practices like meditation, breathwork, or mindfulness can help clear emotional clutter and make room for positive energy. By shifting our internal state from one of resistance to one of openness and gratitude, we align ourselves with the flow of abundance.

Surrendering Control

Letting go also involves surrendering the need to control every aspect of our lives. Many of us try to force outcomes, believing that we need to have all the answers or direct the course of events. However, this need for control often creates tension and blocks the natural flow of opportunities. When we surrender control, we are allowing the universe to work on our behalf. This doesn't mean being passive or complacent—it means taking aligned actions but releasing attachment to the outcome.

In practicing surrender, we develop trust in the process, knowing that what is meant for us will come in its own time and in its own way. This trust opens up the space for new and sometimes unexpected opportunities to enter our lives.

Inviting Abundance and Joy

Abundance is not just about material wealth—it encompasses all aspects of life, from meaningful relationships and personal fulfillment to a sense of purpose and joy. When we invite abundance, we are not just asking for more but creating an internal environment that welcomes growth, prosperity, and joy in all forms. To invite abundance, we must first cultivate a mindset and habits that reflect openness and positivity.

Shifting from Scarcity to Abundance

Many people operate from a mindset of scarcity, believing that resources—whether they be money, love, or opportunities—are limited. This scarcity mindset can keep us trapped in fear, competition, and a constant feeling of lack. To invite abundance, we must shift our perception from scarcity to one of plenty.

This shift begins with gratitude. Gratitude is a powerful tool for rewiring our minds to see abundance in all things, even when it appears scarce. By practicing gratitude daily, we begin to notice the many blessings we already have, which in turn opens us up to receive more. Gratitude signals to the universe that we are content and receptive, which in the Law of Attraction helps attract more of what we appreciate.

Creating an Abundant Environment

Our external environment also plays a key role in inviting abundance. Clutter, disorganization, or being surrounded by things that don't reflect our true desires can block the flow of abundance. A clean, organized space promotes clarity, creativity, and an open mind.

Feng Shui, for instance, is a practice that emphasizes creating an environment conducive to positive energy flow. This principle can be applied by organizing our spaces in a way that promotes peace, flow, and clarity. Surrounding ourselves with beauty, symbols of abundance, and things that bring us joy can also act as a magnet for more positive energy.

Abundance is also reflected in the people we surround ourselves with. If we constantly engage with those who dwell in negativity, complain about life, or focus on scarcity, it's harder to maintain an abundance mindset. Choosing relationships that are uplifting, supportive, and growth-oriented helps to reinforce the energy of abundance in our lives.

The Role of Joy in Manifestation

Joy is one of the most magnetic emotions when it comes to manifestation. When we are joyful, we are in a high vibrational state that attracts positive experiences. Inviting joy into our daily lives opens the door to abundance and opportunity.

Joy can be cultivated in many ways: pursuing hobbies we love, spending time with people who uplift us, or even practicing self-care rituals that make us feel good. Small moments of joy, when consistently experienced, build up over time and lead to an overall state of positivity. The more joy we feel, the more joy we attract, creating a cycle of abundance and fulfillment.

By aligning ourselves with the energy of joy, we naturally become magnets for opportunities, relationships, and experiences that match this high vibration.

Cultivating a Growth Mindset

A growth mindset, as defined by psychologist Carol Dweck, is the belief that our abilities and intelligence can be developed through effort, learning, and perseverance. It stands in contrast to a fixed mindset, where people believe their talents are innate and unchangeable. Cultivating a growth mindset is essential for creating space for new opportunities because it opens us up to continuous learning, self-improvement, and the ability to adapt to change.

Embracing Challenges and Failure

A key element of a growth mindset is the willingness to embrace challenges rather than avoid them. Challenges provide us with opportunities to grow and learn new skills. When we avoid challenges out of fear of failure or discomfort, we limit our potential.

Letting go of the fear of failure is essential to cultivating a growth mindset. Failure is not a reflection of our worth but rather a stepping stone toward success. By reframing failure as a learning experience, we can approach each setback with curiosity and resilience, using it as fuel for future growth. This attitude invites opportunities, as we are more likely to take risks, pursue new endeavors, and keep pushing forward despite obstacles.

Lifelong Learning and Adaptability

Those with a growth mindset understand the value of lifelong learning. They are curious, open to feedback, and constantly seeking ways to improve. By committing to ongoing personal and professional development, we open the door to new opportunities that may not have been available to us otherwise.

Adaptability is another hallmark of a growth mindset. In today's rapidly changing world, those who can adapt to new circumstances, learn new skills, and pivot when necessary are more likely to succeed. Cultivating adaptability allows us to see change as an opportunity rather than a threat.

By embracing learning and adaptability, we position ourselves to take advantage of opportunities that require growth, flexibility, and new knowledge. This mindset also helps us let go of outdated beliefs, habits, or methods that no longer serve us, making room for innovation and progress.

Setting Intentions and Taking Aligned Action

While the Law of Attraction emphasizes the power of thoughts and beliefs, it also requires action. A growth mindset encourages us to take consistent, aligned action toward our goals. Intentions alone are not enough; we must also take the steps necessary to bring those intentions to life.

This doesn't mean forcing outcomes or working tirelessly with no direction. Instead, it means aligning our actions with our desires and taking meaningful steps each day toward our goals. Aligned action stems from clarity, focus, and an understanding of what we want to achieve. When combined with the Law of Attraction, this proactive approach accelerates the manifestation of opportunities and success.

By cultivating a growth mindset, we make room for new challenges, embrace learning, and take action toward our goals. This creates a fertile ground for opportunities to flourish, as we are constantly expanding our skills, knowledge, and perspective.

Thus creating space for new opportunities involves a delicate balance of letting go, inviting abundance, and cultivating a growth mindset. The Law of Attraction teaches us that our thoughts and emotions shape our reality, but we must first let go of what no longer serves us to create room for new experiences. Inviting abundance and joy into our lives opens us up to receiving the blessings that the universe has in store for us.

CHAPTER 9

Living a Life of Freedom

The Benefits of a Let-Go Lifestyle

Staying Open to Life's Flow

Continuing the Journey of Letting Go

Freedom is an elusive concept that can mean different things to different people. For some, freedom is financial independence; for others, it's the ability to travel, make their own decisions, or live without constraints. Yet, at its core, true freedom is often less about external circumstances and more about an internal state of being. It is the result of cultivating a life that allows you to let go of the need for control, embrace the present, and trust the natural flow of life. Living a life of freedom doesn't mean there are no challenges; rather, it's about cultivating the mindset and heartset necessary to handle those challenges with grace.

The Benefits of a Let-Go Lifestyle

1. Emotional Freedom

At the heart of a let-go lifestyle is emotional freedom. When you let go of the things you cannot control, you free yourself from emotional burdens that keep you stuck in a cycle of frustration, anger, or sadness. Emotional freedom is not about becoming indifferent or numb but about developing the resilience to deal with life's challenges without becoming emotionally overwhelmed.

Letting go helps break the habit of dwelling on the past or worrying about the future. It allows you to experience emotions without clinging to them, making room for healing and emotional growth. This freedom can also improve your relationships, as you become more patient and understanding with yourself and others, knowing that everyone is on their own unique journey.

2. Increased Mental Clarity

A mind preoccupied with what it cannot change or with unnecessary worries can become cluttered. Living a let-go lifestyle clears mental space, allowing for greater clarity and focus. When you're not bogged down by regrets, grudges, or anxieties, your mind becomes free to think more creatively, solve problems, and make decisions from a place of calm rather than chaos.

This mental clarity can improve productivity, decision-making, and the overall quality of your daily life. You become more mindful, more present, and more capable of engaging with life as it happens, rather than being lost in a cloud of distractions.

3. Enhanced Relationships

One of the most profound benefits of letting go is how it improves your relationships. When you stop trying to control others or hold onto unrealistic expectations, you create space for authentic connections. A let-go lifestyle teaches you to embrace people for who they are, rather than who you want them to be. This shift leads to deeper, more meaningful relationships built on trust and mutual respect.

Letting go also frees you from the need to constantly prove yourself to others. When you're no longer seeking validation, you can be more honest, vulnerable, and authentic in your interactions. This vulnerability fosters stronger connections because it allows others to see and accept the real you.

4. Reduced Stress and Anxiety

Stress often comes from the pressure to control things that are outside our control. Whether it's trying to control outcomes, people's opinions, or future events, this desire to dictate the course of life leads to anxiety and tension. A let-go lifestyle helps you release the need for control and embrace uncertainty, thereby reducing the stress that comes from holding on too tightly to expectations.

By letting go, you cultivate a sense of inner peace that comes from knowing that you are not responsible for controlling everything. This mindset allows you to approach challenges with more calm and grace, accepting that some things are beyond your control, and that's okay.

5. Increased Opportunities for Growth

When you hold on to the familiar out of fear or resistance to change, you block new opportunities from coming into your life. A let-go lifestyle encourages you to release your grip on what no longer serves you, opening up space for new possibilities. Whether it's in your career, relationships, or personal development, letting go allows you to move forward rather than staying stuck.

This openness to growth is transformative. It gives you the courage to step outside your comfort zone, take risks, and explore new paths. You begin to see challenges not as obstacles but as opportunities for learning and self-discovery.

Staying Open to Life's Flow

1. Embracing Uncertainty

Life is inherently unpredictable. While we often seek to establish control through routines, plans, and expectations, the reality is that uncertainty is an inescapable part of life. Staying open to life's flow means learning to embrace the unknown and trusting that even when things don't go according to plan, there is value in the unfolding journey.

By embracing uncertainty, you free yourself from the fear of the unknown. This freedom allows you to approach life with curiosity and openness rather than resistance. When you're open to life's flow, you begin to see that every detour, every unexpected twist, holds potential for growth and discovery.

2. Cultivating Flexibility

Being open to life's flow requires flexibility, both mentally and emotionally. Flexibility means being able to adapt to change, adjust your expectations, and respond to life's challenges with resilience. It means being willing to let go of rigid ideas, whether they're about how your life should unfold, how other people should behave, or how you should feel.

Cultivating flexibility doesn't mean you become passive or directionless. Instead, it's about learning to balance intention with surrender. You set goals and work toward them, but you're also willing to adjust your course when life presents something unexpected.

3. Practicing Mindfulness

Staying open to life's flow also means being present in the moment. When you're preoccupied with the past or the future, you're not truly open to what life is offering right now. Practicing mindfulness allows you to engage with the present moment, to experience it fully without judgment or expectation.

Mindfulness teaches you to let go of the need for constant control. It invites you to experience life as it is, rather than how you think it should be. By focusing on the present, you become more attuned to life's natural rhythm, allowing you to flow with it rather than against it.

4. Trusting the Process

At the core of staying open to life's flow is trust—trust in yourself, trust in the process, and trust that life is unfolding exactly as it should. Trusting the process doesn't mean everything will always go smoothly or according to plan. It means believing that, no matter what happens, you have the inner strength and wisdom to navigate it.

This trust frees you from the constant need to control or predict the future. It allows you to take action without attachment to specific outcomes, knowing that even when things don't turn out as expected, there is a reason, a lesson, or a hidden opportunity.

Continuing the Journey of Letting Go

1. Letting Go as a Lifelong Practice

The journey of letting go is not a one-time event but a lifelong practice. It's an ongoing process of releasing what no longer serves you—whether it's negative thoughts, toxic relationships, outdated beliefs, or past experiences. Each time you let go, you create space for new opportunities, new insights, and new growth.

As you continue this journey, you will find that letting go becomes easier and more natural. With each experience, you gain greater clarity and wisdom, allowing you to live with more freedom, peace, and joy. It's a journey that deepens with time, offering new layers of understanding as you grow and evolve.

2. Overcoming Setbacks and Resistance

Even when you commit to a let-go lifestyle, there will be times when you encounter resistance. Letting go can be difficult, especially when it involves things we are deeply attached to, such as identities, relationships, or long-held beliefs. In these moments, it's important to recognize that setbacks are part of the process.

Overcoming resistance involves practicing patience and self-compassion. It means acknowledging the difficulty of letting go without judging yourself for struggling. The more you practice, the more you develop the inner resilience to face these challenges with grace and determination.

3. Celebrating Small Wins

One of the keys to continuing the journey of letting go is to celebrate your progress, no matter how small it may seem. Each time you release something that no longer serves you, take a moment to recognize the growth that has occurred. These small wins are the building blocks of a freer, more authentic life.

By celebrating your progress, you reinforce the positive changes you're making, which in turn encourages you to keep going. Over time, these small wins accumulate, leading to profound transformation and a deeper sense of freedom.

4. Living with Intention

Continuing the journey of letting go also involves living with intention. This means being clear about what you value, what you want to prioritize in your life, and what you're willing to release in order to stay true to those values. Living with intention helps you make conscious choices about where you direct your energy and attention.

When you live with intention, you're less likely to hold onto things that no longer serve you. Instead, you focus on what truly matters, allowing you to live a life of greater meaning, purpose, and fulfillment.

5. Expanding Your Capacity for Love and Compassion

As you continue to let go, you expand your capacity for love and compassion—both for yourself and for others. Letting go of grudges, resentments, and unrealistic expectations allows you to cultivate a more open heart. This openness enables you to give and receive love more freely, without the fear of being hurt or disappointed.

Compassion also becomes a guiding force in your life. When you stop holding onto judgments, you create space for empathy and understanding. This compassion extends not only to others but also to yourself, allowing you to navigate life's ups and downs with greater kindness and acceptance.

CONCLUSION

Reflecting on Your Journey

Embracing the Power of Letting Go

Moving Forward with Confidence

As you reflect on your journey through this book, you've taken a courageous step toward transforming your life. Letting go is not merely a process; it's a profound act of self-liberation. Each chapter has encouraged you to peel back the layers of attachment, fear, and doubt, exposing the limitless potential within. By embracing the power of letting go, you're no longer bound by the chains of the past or the uncertainty of the future. Instead, you stand firmly in the present, where true freedom resides.

Embracing the Power of Letting Go

The act of letting go is a powerful declaration that you trust in the flow of life. It is a surrender not to defeat, but to the beauty of growth, change, and renewal. By releasing what no longer serves you—be it limiting beliefs, toxic relationships, or past hurts—you make room for new possibilities. Letting go isn't about forgetting; it's about finding peace with what has been, so you can fully embrace what is and what will be.

You now possess the tools and understanding to walk this path with grace, knowing that your worth and happiness aren't tied to what you hold onto but to your willingness to evolve.

Moving Forward with Confidence

Moving forward, you are equipped with the confidence to face whatever life brings your way. The power of letting go has strengthened your resilience, broadened your perspective, and deepened your sense of self. With each step, trust that you are walking in alignment with your highest self, capable of navigating life's complexities with calm assurance. This newfound freedom empowers you to create space for joy, abundance, and purpose.

As you continue your journey, remember: the act of letting go is ongoing. It's a practice that will serve you throughout your life. So, carry with you the lessons learned, the wisdom gained, and the knowledge

that you have the strength to let go,
and in doing so, to truly live.

www.ingramcontent.com/pod-product-compliance
Lightning Source LLC
Chambersburg PA
CBHW051607250726

48653CB00004BA/1379